CW00435450

Ketogenic Diet
For Women
Over 50

50 Recipes For Losing Weight
And Reshaping Your Body

Tiffany Johnson

TABLE OF CONTENTS

INTRODUCTION

Over the age of 50, it is hard to maintain good health and shed extra weight, especially for women. Either they are experiencing menopause, having more time to eat and socializing, losing weight after 50 is not easy.

The ketogenic diet provides the body with premium fuel in the form of fats that make you fitter and younger with the energy of a twenty-year-old, and the best part, it lasts longer than carb fuel.

By following the ketogenic diet, you can lose all the unwanted weight without ever stepping foot in a gym, without any meal portion control or counting calories. The ketogenic diet has proven to work for people with all types of background and health issues like having blood sugar issues, obesity, post-pregnancy, people having food addictions, suffering from emotional eating, etc.

Adaptation to ketosis can be tough, and you will need time to adjust to the changes. It is normal, and everyone faces troubles in adapting to any new dietary plan. However, here are some steps to help you in transiting into the ketogenic diet plan perfectly. Just remember that it does require time, and you will have to give yourself a little space to adjust to the restrictions. It won't happen overnight, so don't be disheartened and stay motivated!

The most basic mistake that many keto dieters make is that they don't gain enough knowledge before starting the diet. Therefore, the most important step is to learn the small differences that make a huge difference. Understand what keto-friendly foods are what foods are not meant for ketosis at all. For example, a lot of apple does not eat an apple because it has many carbs. However, if you have a medium or a small-sized apple, then you are good to have it. As long as it remains within your carb limit, it is keto-friendly. You can also eat an apple a day (depending on the size), but you need to remember ketosis's essence and take your carbs from energetic sources like protein and healthy fats. Once you can understand the difference between non-keto and keto-friendly foods, you will notice that ketosis is not that tough after all.

The best way to transit in ketosis is to keep track of your carbs. This might seem annoying at first, but you will gradually see how helpful it is, and you will eventually understand the importance of calculating the net carbs per day. It is extremely crucial, and usually, people overlook this issue quite easily. However, if you want to settle into ketosis perfectly, it is best to keep track of your net carbs.

Mindful eating is a very important step towards transition into ketosis. Your caloric intake has a huge impact on your weight loss. The more calories you take, the harder it gets to lose the stubborn, stored fat. A keto calculator can be extremely helpful in this matter, though. You can calculate your caloric intake on the go and limit your food intake accordingly. Also, before you pick something to eat, you can instantly calculate the calories you will take. This is known as mindful eating, knowing what you are eating and how it will affect you.

Ketosis is all about gaining knowledge and getting into the habit of mindful eating. Once you know what you are eating and how much it has to offer to you, you will gradually see major changes in your overall diet routine. You will also find yourself adjusting to ketosis much easier.

BREAKFAST

1. Veggie Frittata

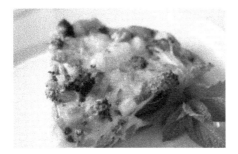

Preparation Time: 10 minutes

Cooking Time: 4 hours

Servings: 4

Ingredients:

- 6 eggs
- 2 tsp.... Italian seasoning
- 1/4 cup cherry tomatoes, sliced
- 4 oz... mushrooms, sliced
- 1/2 cup cheese, shredded
- Pepper and salt

Directions:

1. Spray slow cooker from inside with cooking spray.
2. Spray medium pan with cooking spray and heat over medium heat.
3. Add mushrooms and cherry tomatoes to the pan and cook until softened.
4. Transfer vegetables to the slow cooker.

5. In a bowl, whisk together eggs, cheese, pepper, and salt.

6. Whisk egg mixture into the slow cooker.

7. Cover and cook on low.

8. Slice and serve.

Nutrition: Calories 167 Fat 12 g Carbs 2.3 g Sugar 1.6 g Protein 12.8 g Cholesterol 262 mg

2. Feta Spinach Quiche

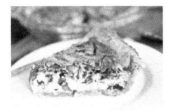

Preparation Time: 10 minutes

Cooking Time: 8 hours

Servings: 6

Ingredients:

- 8 eggs
- 3/4 cup feta cheese, crumbled
- 3/4 cup parmesan cheese, shredded
- 2 cups spinach, chopped
- 2 cups unsweetened coconut milk
- Pepper and salt

Directions:

1. Spray slow cooker from inside with cooking spray.
2. In a bowl, whisk together eggs and coconut milk.
3. Add spinach, parmesan cheese, feta cheese, and salt and stir to combine.
4. Pour egg mixture into the slow cooker.
5. Cover and cook on low.
6. Slice and serve.

Nutrition: Calories 375 Fat 32.6 g Carbs 6.5 g Sugar 3.9 g Protein 17.2 g Cholesterol 245 mg

3. Kalua Pork with Cabbage

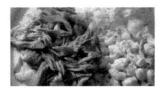

Preparation Time: 10 minutes

Cooking Time: 9 hours

Servings: 12

Ingredients:

- 1 medium cabbage head, chopped
- 3 lbs. pork shoulder butt roast, trimmed
- 7 bacon slices
- 1 tbsp... sea salt

Directions:

1. Place 4 bacon slices into the bottom of slow cooker.
2. Spread pork roast on top of bacon slices and season with salt.
3. Arrange remaining bacon slices on top of pork roast layer.
4. Cover and cook on low until meat is tender.
5. Add chopped cabbage. Cover again and cook on low
6. Detach pork from slow cooker and shred.
7. \take back the shredded pork to the slow cooker and stir well.
8. Serve warm and enjoy.

Nutrition: Calories 264 Fat 18.4 g Carbs 4.4 g Sugar 2.4 g Protein 20.5 g Cholesterol 71 mg

4. Creamy Pork Chops

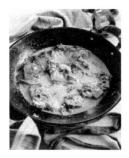

Preparation Time: 10 minutes

Cooking Time: 6 hours

Servings: 4

Ingredients:

- 4 boneless pork chops
- 1/2 cup chicken stock
- 1 oz... dry ranch dressing
- 10.5 oz... chicken soup
- 3 garlic cloves, minced
- Pepper

Directions:

1. Season pork chops with pepper and place in slow cooker.
2. In a bowl, mix together chicken soup, ranch dressing, stock, and garlic.
3. Pour chicken soup mixture over top of pork chops.
4. Cover and cook on low.
5. Serve hot and enjoy.

Nutrition: Calories 280 Fat 15.1 g Carbs 4.7 g Sugar 1 g Protein 29.1 g Cholesterol 64 mg

LUNCH

5. Lunch Chicken Wraps

Preparation time: 18 minutes

Cooking time: 6 hours

Servings: 6

Ingredients:

- 6 tortillas
- 3 tablespoon Caesar dressing
- 1-pound chicken breast
- 1/2 cup lettuce
- cup water
- 1 oz. bay leaf
- 1 teaspoon salt
- 1 teaspoon ground pepper
- 1 teaspoon coriander
- 4 oz. Feta cheese

Directions:

1. Put the chicken breast in the slow cooker.
2. Sprinkle the meat with the bay leaf, salt, ground pepper, and coriander.
3. Add water and cook the chicken breast for 6 hours on LOW.
4. Then remove the cooked chicken from the slow cooker and shred it with a fork.
5. Chop the lettuce roughly.

6. Then chop Feta cheese. Combine the chopped Ingredients: together and add the shredded chicken breast and Caesar dressing.

7. Mix everything together well. After this, spread the tortillas with the shredded chicken mixture and wrap them. Enjoy!

Nutrition: Calories 376 Fat 18.5 Fiber 3 Carbs 2.3, Protein 23

6. Butternut Squash Soup

Preparation time: 10 minutes

Cooking time: 8 hours

Servings: 9

Ingredients:

- 2-pound butternut squash
- 4 teaspoon minced garlic
- 1/2 cup onion, chopped
- teaspoon salt
- 1/4 teaspoon ground nutmeg
- 1 teaspoon ground black pepper
- 8 cups chicken stock
- 1 tablespoon fresh parsley

Directions:

1. Peel the butternut squash and cut it into the chunks.
2. Toss the butternut squash in the slow cooker.
3. Add chopped onion, minced garlic, and chicken stock.
4. Close the slow cooker lid and cook the soup for 8 hours on LOW.
5. Meanwhile, combine the ground black pepper, ground nutmeg, and salt together.
6. Chop the fresh parsley.
7. When the time is done, remove the soup from the slow cooker and blend it with a blender until you get a creamy soup.
8. Sprinkle the soup with the spice mixture and add chopped parsley. Serve the soup warm. Enjoy!

Nutrition: Calories 129 Fat 2.7 Fiber 2 Carbs 2.85 Protein 7

7. Eggplant Bacon Wraps

Preparation time: 17 minutes

Cooking time: 5 hours

Servings: 6

Ingredients:

- 10 oz. eggplant, sliced into rounds
- 5 oz. halloumi cheese
- 1 teaspoon minced garlic
- 3 oz. bacon, chopped
- 1/2 teaspoon ground black pepper
- 1 teaspoon salt
- 1 teaspoon paprika
- 1 tomato

Directions:

1. Rub the eggplant slices with the ground black pepper, salt, and paprika.
2. Slice halloumi cheese and tomato.
3. Combine the chopped bacon and minced garlic together.
4. Place the sliced eggplants in the slow cooker. Cook the eggplant on HIGH for 1 hour.
5. Chill the eggplant. Place the sliced tomato and cheese on the eggplant slices.
6. Add the chopped bacon mixture and roll up tightly.
7. Secure the eggplants with the toothpicks and return the eggplant wraps back into the slow cookies. Cook the dish on HIGH for 4 hours more.

8. When the dish is done, serve it immediately. Enjoy!

Nutrition: Calories 131, Fat 9.4, Fiber 2, Carbs 1.25, Protein 6

8. Mexican Warm Salad

Preparation time: 26 minutes

Cooking time: 10 hours

Servings: 10

Ingredients:

- 1cup black beans
- 1cup sweet corn, frozen
- 3 tomatoes
- 1/2 cup fresh dill
- chili pepper
- 7 oz. chicken fillet
- 5 oz. Cheddar cheese
- 4tablespoons mayonnaise
- 1teaspoon minced garlic
- 1cup lettuce
- 5cups chicken stock
- 1cucumber

Directions:

1. Put the chicken fillet, sweet corn, black beans, and chicken stock in the slow cooker.
2. Close the slow cooker lid and cook the mixture on LOW for 10 hours.
3. When the time is done remove the mixture from the slow cooker.
4. Shred the chicken fillet with 2 forks. Chill the mixture until room temperature.

5. Chop the lettuce roughly. Chop the cucumber and tomatoes.

6. Place the lettuce, cucumber, and tomatoes on a large serving plate.

7. After this, shred Cheddar cheese and chop the chili pepper.

8. Add the chili pepper to the serving plate too.

9. After this, add the chicken mixture on the top of the salad.

10. Sprinkle the salad with the mayonnaise, minced garlic, and shredded cheese. Enjoy the salad immediately.

Nutrition: Calories 182, Fat 7.8, Fiber 2, Carbs 1.6, Protein 9

9. Hot Chorizo Salad

Preparation time: 20 minutes

Cooking time: 4 hours 30 minutes

Servings: 6

Ingredients:

- 8 oz. chorizo
- 1teaspoon olive oil
- 1teaspoon cayenne pepper
- 1teaspoon chili flakes
- 1teaspoon ground black pepper
- 1teaspoon onion powder
- 2garlic cloves
- 3tomatoes
- 1cup lettuce
- 1cup fresh dill
- 1teaspoon oregano
- 3tablespoons crushed cashews

Directions:

1. Chop the chorizo sausages roughly and place them in the slow cooker.
2. Cook the sausages for 4 hours on HIGH.
3. Meanwhile, combine the cayenne pepper, chili flakes, ground black pepper, and onion powder together in a shallow bowl.
4. Chop the tomatoes roughly and add them to the slow cooker after 4 hours. Cook the mixture for 30 minutes more on HIGH.

5. Chop the fresh dill and combine it with oregano.

6. When the chorizo sausage mixture is cooked, place it in a serving bowl. Tear the lettuce and add it in the bowl too.

7. After this, peel the garlic cloves and slice them.

8. Add the sliced garlic cloves in the salad bowl too.

9. Then sprinkle the salad with the spice mixture, olive oil, fresh dill mixture, and crush cashew. Mix the salad carefully. Enjoy!

Nutrition: Calories 249, Fat 19.8, Fiber 2, Carbs 1.69, Protein 11

10. Stuffed Eggplants

Preparation time: 20 minutes

Cooking time: 8 hours

Servings: 4

Ingredients:

- 4medium eggplants
- 1cup rice, half cooked
- 1/2cup chicken stock
- 1teaspoon salt
- 1teaspoon paprika
- 1/2cup fresh cilantro
- 3tablespoons tomato sauce
- 1teaspoon olive oil

Directions:

1. Wash the eggplants carefully and remove the flesh from them.
2. Then combine the rice with the salt, paprika, and tomato sauce.
3. Chop the fresh cilantro and add it to the rice mixture.
4. Then fill the prepared eggplants with the rice mixture.
5. Pour the chicken stock and olive oil in the slow cooker.
6. Add the stuffed eggplants and close the slow cooker lid.
7. Cook the dish on LOW for 8 hours. When the eggplants are done, chill them little and serve immediately. Enjoy!

Nutrition: Calories 277, Fat 9.1, Fiber 24, Carbs 1.92, Protein 11

11. Light Lunch Quiche

Preparation time: 21 minutes

Cooking time: 4 hours 25 minutes

Servings: 7

Ingredients:

- 7oz. pie crust
- 1/4cup broccoli
- 1/3cup sweet peas
- 1/4cup heavy cream
- 2tablespoons flour
- 3eggs
- 4oz. Romano cheese, shredded
- 1teaspoon cilantro
- 1teaspoon salt
- 1/4cup spinach
- 1tomato

Directions:

1. Cover the inside of the slow cooker bowl with parchment.
2. Put the pie crust inside and flatten it well with your fingertips.
3. Chop the broccoli and combine it with sweet peas. Combine the heavy cream, flour, cilantro, and salt together. Stir the liquid until smooth.
4. Then beat the eggs into the heavy cream liquid and mix it with a hand mixer. When you get a smooth mix, combine it with the broccoli.

5. Chop the spinach and add it to the mix. Chop the tomato and add it to the mix too. Pour the prepared mixture into the pie crust slowly.

6. Close the slow cooker lid and cook the quiche for 4 hours on HIGH.

7. After 4 hours, sprinkle the quiche surface with the shredded cheese and cook the dish for 25 minutes more. Serve the prepared quiche! Enjoy!

Nutrition: Calories 287, Fat 18.8, Fiber 1, Carbs 1.1, Protein 11

12. Chicken Open Sandwich

Preparation time: 15 minutes

Cooking time: 8 hours

Servings: 4

Ingredients:

- 7oz. chicken fillet
- 1teaspoon cayenne pepper
- 5oz. mashed potato, cooked
- 6tablespoons chicken gravy
- 4slices French bread, toasted
- 2teaspoons mayo
- 1cup water

Directions:

1. Put the chicken fillet in the slow cooker and sprinkle it with the cayenne pepper.
2. Add water and chicken gravy. Close the slow cooker lid and cook the chicken for 8 hours on LOW. Then combine the mashed potato with the mayo sauce.
3. Spread toasted French bread with the mashed potato mixture.
4. When the chicken is cooked, cut it into the strips and combine with the remaining gravy from the slow cooker.
5. Place the chicken strips over the mashed potato. Enjoy the open sandwich warm!

Nutrition: Calories 314, Fat 9.7, Fiber 3, Carbs 4.1, Protein 12

13. Onion Lunch Muffins

Preparation time: 15 minutes

Cooking time: 8 hours

Servings: 7

Ingredients:

- 1egg
- 5tablespoons butter, melted
- 1cup flour
- 1/2cup milk
- 1teaspoon baking soda
- 1cup onion, chopped
- 1teaspoon cilantro
- 1/2teaspoon sage
- 1teaspoon apple cider vinegar
- 2cup water
- 1tablespoon chives
- 1teaspoon olive oil

Directions:

1. Beat the egg in the bowl and add melted butter.
2. Add the flour, baking soda, chopped onion, milk, sage, apple cider vinegar, cilantro, and chives. Knead into a dough.
3. After this, spray a muffin form with the olive oil inside. Fill the 1/2 part of every muffin form and place them in the glass jars.
4. After this, pour water in the slow cooker vessel.
5. Place the glass jars with muffins in the slow cooker and close the lid.

6. Cook the muffins for 8 hours on LOW.

7. Check if the muffins are cooked with the help of the toothpick and remove them from the slow cooker. Enjoy the dish warm!

Nutrition: Calories 180, Fat 11, Fiber 1, Carbs 1.28, Protein 4

DINNER

14. Lemon Dill Halibut

Preparation Time: 5 minutes

Cooking Time: 2 hours

Servings: 6

Ingredients:

- 12-ounce wild-caught halibut fillet
- 1teaspoon salt
- 1/2teaspoon ground black pepper
- 11/2 teaspoon dried dill
- 1tablespoon fresh lemon juice
- 3tablespoons avocado oil

Directions:

1. Cut an 18-inch piece of aluminum foil, place halibut fillet in the middle and then season with salt and black pepper.

2. Whisk together remaining ingredients, drizzle this mixture over halibut, then crimp the edges of foil and place it into a 6-quart slow cooker.

3. Plug in the slow cooker, shut with lid and cook for 1 hour and 30 minutes or 2 hours at high heat setting or until cooked through.

4. When done, carefully open the crimped edges and check the fish, it should be tender and flaky.

5. Serve straightaway.

Nutrition: Calories: 312 Fat: 15 g Protein: 13.8 g Carbs: 0 g Fiber: 7 g Sugar: 0 g

15. Coconut Cilantro Curry Shrimp

Preparation Time: 5 minutes

Cooking Time: 2 hours

Servings: 4

Ingredients:

- 1pound wild-caught shrimp, peeled and deveined
- 21/2teaspoon lemon garlic seasoning
- 2tablespoons red curry paste
- 4tablespoons chopped cilantro
- 30ounces coconut milk, unsweetened
- 16ounces water

Directions:

1. Whisk together all the ingredients except for shrimps and 2 tablespoons cilantro and add to a 4-quart slow cooker.

2. Plug in the slow cooker, shut with lid and cook for 2 hours at high heat setting or 4 hours at low heat setting.

3. Then add shrimps, toss until evenly coated and cook for 20 to 30 minutes at high heat settings or until shrimps are pink.

4. Garnish shrimps with remaining cilantro and serve.

Nutrition: Calories: 213 Fat: 12 g Protein: 15 g Carbs: 1.9 g Fiber: 7 g Sugar: 1.4 g

16. Shrimp in Marinara Sauce

Preparation Time: 5 minutes

Cooking Time: 5 hours

Servings: 5

Ingredients:

- 1pound cooked wild-caught shrimps, peeled and deveined
- 14.5ounce crushed tomatoes
- 1/2teaspoon minced garlic
- 1teaspoon salt
- 1/2teaspoon seasoned salt
- 1/4teaspoon ground black pepper
- 1/2teaspoon crushed red pepper flakes
- 1/2teaspoon dried basil
- 1/2teaspoon dried oregano
- 1/2tablespoons avocado oil
- 6-ounce chicken broth
- 2tablespoon minced parsley
- 1/2cup grated Parmesan cheese

Directions:

1. Place all the ingredients except for shrimps, parsley, and cheese in a 4-quart slow cooker and stir well.
2. Then plug in the slow cooker, shut with lid and cook for 4 to 5 hours at low heat setting.
3. Then add shrimps and parsley, stir until mixed and cook for 10 minutes at high heat setting.
4. Garnish shrimps with cheese and serve.

Nutrition: Calories: 213 Fat: 12 g Protein: 15 g Carbs: 3.9 g Fiber: 7 g Sugar: 3.6 g

17. Garlic Shrimp

Preparation Time: 5 minutes

Cooking Time: 5 hours

Servings: 5

Ingredients:

- For the Garlic Shrimp:
- 11/2 pounds large wild-caught shrimp, peeled and deveined
- 1/4teaspoon ground black pepper
- 1/8teaspoon ground cayenne pepper
- 2 1/2teaspoons minced garlic
- 1/4cup avocado oil
- 4tablespoons unsalted butter
- For the Seasoning:
- 1teaspoon onion powder
- 1tablespoon garlic powder
- 1tablespoon salt
- 2teaspoons ground black pepper
- 1tablespoon paprika
- 1teaspoon cayenne pepper
- 1teaspoon dried oregano
- 1teaspoon dried thyme

Directions:

1. Stir together all the ingredients for seasoning, garlic, oil, and butter and add to a 4-quart slow cooker.

2. Plug in the slow cooker, shut with lid and cook for 25 to 30 minutes at high heat setting or until cooked.

3. Then add shrimps, toss until evenly coated and continue cooking for 20 to 30 minutes at high heat setting or until shrimps are pink.

4. When done, transfer shrimps to a serving plate, top with sauce and serve.

Nutrition: Calories: 227 Fat: 13 g Protein: 21 g Carbs: 1.2 g Fiber: 7 g Sugar: 5 g

18. Poached Salmon

Preparation Time: 5 minutes

Cooking Time: 3 hours

Servings: 4

Ingredients:

- 4steaks of wild-caught salmon
- 1medium white onion, peeled and sliced
- 2teaspoons minced garlic
- 1/2teaspoon salt
- 1/8teaspoon ground white pepper
- 1/2teaspoon dried dill weed
- 2tablespoons avocado oil
- 2tablespoons unsalted butter
- 2tablespoons lemon juice
- 1cup water

Directions:

1. Place butter in a 4-quart slow cooker, then add salmon and drizzle with oil.
2. Place remaining ingredients in a medium saucepan, stir until mixed and bring the mixture to boil over high heat.
3. Then pour this mixture all over salmon and shut with lid.
4. Plug in the slow cooker and cook salmon for 3 hours and 30 minutes at low heat setting or until salmon is tender.
5. Serve straightaway.

Nutrition: Calories: 338 Fat: 11 g Protein: 13 g Carbs: 2.8 g Fiber: 7 g Sugar: 1.2 g

19. Lemon Pepper Tilapia

Preparation Time: 5 minutes

Cooking Time: 3 hours

Servings: 6

Ingredients:

- 6 wild-caught Tilapia fillets
- 4teaspoons lemon-pepper seasoning, divided
- 6tablespoons unsalted butter, divided
- 1/2cup lemon juice, fresh

Directions:

1. Cut a large piece of aluminum foil for each fillet and then arrange them on a clean working space.

2. Place each fillet in the middle of the foil, then season with lemon-pepper seasoning, drizzle with lemon juice and top with 1 tablespoon butter.

3. Gently crimp the edges of foil to form a packet and place it into a 6-quart slow cooker.

4. Plug in the slow cooker, shut with lid and cook for 3 hours at high heat setting or until cooked through.

5. When done, carefully remove packets from the slow cooker and open the crimped edges and check the fish, it should be tender and flaky.

6. Serve straightaway.

Nutrition: Calories: 321 Fat: 10 g Protein: 21 g Carbs: 1.2 g Fiber: 7 g Sugar: 1.8 g

20. Clam Chowder

Preparation Time: 5 minutes

Cooking Time: 6 hours

Servings: 6

Ingredients:

- 20-ounce wild-caught baby clams, with juice
- 1/2cup chopped scallion
- 1/2cup chopped celery
- 1teaspoon salt
- 1teaspoon ground black pepper
- 1teaspoon dried thyme
- 1tablespoon avocado oil
- 2cups coconut cream, full-fat
- 2cups chicken broth

Directions:

1. Grease a 6-quart slow cooker with oil, then add ingredients and stir until mixed.
2. Plug in the slow cooker, shut with lid and cook for 4 to 6 hours at low heat setting or until cooked through.
3. Serve straightaway.

Nutrition: Calories: 190 Fat: 14 g Protein: 12 g Carbs: 4.1 g Fiber: 17 g Sugar: 3.9 g

21. Soy-Ginger Steamed Pompano

Preparation Time: 5 minutes

Cooking Time: 1 hour

Servings: 6

Ingredients:

- 1wild-caught whole pompano, gutted and scaled
- 1bunch scallion, diced
- 1 bunch cilantro, chopped
- 3teaspoons minced garlic
- 1tablespoon grated ginger
- 1tablespoon swerve sweetener
- 1/4cup soy sauce
- 1/4 cup white wine
- 1/4 cup sesame oil

Directions:

1. Place scallions in a 6-quart slow cooker and top with fish.
2. Whisk together remaining ingredients, except for cilantro, and pour the mixture all over the fish.
3. Plug in the slow cooker, shut with lid and cook for 1 hour at high heat setting or until cooked through.
4. Garnish with cilantro and serve.

Nutrition: Calories: 129 Fat: 13 g Protein: 18 g Carbs: 4 g Fiber: 17 g Sugar: 3.1 g

22. Vietnamese Braised Catfish

Preparation Time: 5 minutes

Cooking Time: 6 hours

Servings: 3

Ingredients:

- 1fillet of wild-caught catfish, cut into bite-size pieces
- 1scallion, chopped
- 3red chilies, chopped
- 1tablespoon grated ginger
- 1/2cup swerve sweetener
- 2tablespoons avocado oil
- 1/4cup fish sauce, unsweetened

Directions:

1. Place a small saucepan over medium heat, add sweetener and cook until it melts.
2. Then add scallion, chilies, ginger and fish sauce and stir until mixed.
3. Transfer this mixture in a 4-quart slow cooker, add fish and toss until coated.
4. Plug in the slow cooker, shut with lid and cook for 6 hours at low heat setting until cooked.
5. Drizzle with avocado oil and serve straightaway.

Nutrition: Calories: 156 Fat: 21 g Protein: 19 g Carbs: 0.2 g Fiber: 17 g Sugar: 0.1 g

23. Chili Prawns

Preparation Time: 5 minutes

Cooking Time: 1 hour

Servings: 6

Ingredients:

- 18-ounce wild-caught prawns, shell-on
- 1/2cup sliced scallions
- 1thumb-sized ginger, minced
- 1bulb. of garlic, peeled and minced
- 1tablespoon swerve sweetener
- 2tablespoons apple cider vinegar
- 2tablespoons Sambal Oelek
- 1tablespoon fish sauce, unsweetened
- 4tablespoons sesame oil
- 1/2cup tomato ketchup, keto and unsweetened
- 1egg, beaten

Directions:

1. Place all the ingredients, except for prawns, oil, and egg in a 6-quart slow cooker and stir until mixed.
2. Plug in the slow cooker, shut with lid and cook for 1 hour at high heat setting.
3. Then add prawns and continue cooking for 15 minutes at high heat setting or until prawns turn pink.
4. Stir in oil and egg and cook for 10 minutes.
5. Drizzle with more fish sauce and serve.

Nutrition: Calories: 154 Fat: 13 g Protein: 15 g Carbs: 3.6 g Fiber: 17 g Sugar: 1.7 g

24. Tuna Salpicao

Preparation Time: 5 minutes

Cooking Time: 3 hours

Servings: 2

Ingredients:

- 8ounce cooked wild-caught tuna, cut into inch cubes
- 4jalapeno peppers, chopped
- 5red chili, chopped
- 1bulb. of garlic, peeled and minced
- 1teaspoon salt
- 1teaspoon ground black pepper
- 1cup avocado oil

Directions:

1. Place all the ingredients except for tuna in a 4-quart slow cooker and stir until mixed.

2. Plug in the slow cooker, shut with lid and cook for 4 hours at low heat setting.

3. Then add tuna and continue cooking for 10 minutes at high heat setting.

4. Serve straightaway.

Nutrition: Calories: 154 Fat: 13 g Protein: 15 g Carbs: 1.8 g Fiber: 17 g Sugar: 1.0 g

25. Soy-Ginger Braised Squid

Preparation Time: 5 minutes

Cooking Time: 8 hours

Servings: 6

Ingredients:

- 18-ounce wild-caught squid, cut into rings
- 2scallions, chopped
- 2bay leaves
- 1tablespoon grated ginger
- 1bulb. of garlic, peeled and minced
- 1/2cup swerve sweetener
- 1/4cup soy sauce
- 1/4cup oyster sauce
- 1/4cup avocado oil
- 1/4cup white wine

Directions:

1. Plug in a 6-quart slow cooker, add all the ingredients and stir until mixed.
2. Shut with lid and cook for 8 hours at low heat setting or until cooked through.
3. Serve straightaway.

Nutrition: Calories: 154 Fat: 13 g Protein: 15 g Carbs: 3.4 g Fiber: 17 g Sugar: 1.9 g

26. Sea Bass in Coconut Cream Sauce

Preparation Time: 5 minutes

Cooking Time: 1 hour

Servings: 3

Ingredients:

- 18-ounce wild-caught sea bass
- 5jalapeno peppers
- 4stalks of bock Choy
- 2stalks of scallions, sliced
- 1tablespoon grated ginger
- 11/2 teaspoon salt
- 1tablespoon fish sauce, unsweetened
- 2cups coconut cream

Directions:

1. Stir together all the ingredients except for bok choy and fish in a bowl and add this mixture in a 6-quarts slow cooker.

2. Plug in the slow cooker, then add fish, top with bok choy and shut with lid.

3. Cook sea bass for 1 hour and 30 minutes or until cooked.

4. Serve straightaway.

Nutrition: Calories: 315 Fat: 17 g Protein: 15 g Carbs: 2.4 g Fiber: 17 g Sugar: 3.2 g

27. Beef & Pumpkin Stew

Preparation Time: 5 minutes

Cooking Time: 4 hours

Servings: 4

Ingredients:

- Teaspoon sage
- teaspoon mixed herbs
- Tablespoons rosemary
- Tablespoons thyme
- 6 tablespoons coconut oil
- 200g pumpkin
- 300g stewing steak
- Salt & pepper, to taste

Directions:

1. Trim off every excess fat from the stewing steak, then transfer it into the crockpot.
2. Season the steak with half of the coconut oil then and in the salt & pepper.
3. Cover the crockpot, then cook on high setting for 1 hour.
4. Remove the steak from the crockpot to a serving platter alongside all the remaining seasoning and coconut oil.
5. Mix everything, then transfer back into the crockpot with the pumpkin and cook for 3 hours on a low setting.
6. Serve with fresh mixed herbs and enjoy.

Nutrition: Calories: 324 Carbs: 3.7g Fat: 11g Protein: 23g

SNACKS RECIPES

28. Bacon Chive Dip

Preparation Time: 5 minutes

Cooking Time: 10 minutes

Servings: 4

Ingredients:

- 1-pound bacon
- 8 ounces' cream cheese
- 1/2 cup ranch dressing
- 1/2 cup sour cream
- 1/2 cup Chicken Broth (see recipe in Chapter 3)
- 1 cup shredded sharp cheddar cheese
- 1/4 cup fresh chopped chives

Directions:

1. Chop bacon into small pieces. Press the Sauté button. Press the Adjust button to set heat to less. Add bacon to Instant Pot. Once fat begins to render from bacon, after about 5 minutes, press the Cancel button.

2. Press the Sauté button and then press the Adjust button to set heat to Normal. Continue cooking bacon until crisp. When bacon is finished, remove and place on paper towel.

3. Press the Cancel button. Add cream cheese, ranch, sour cream, broth, and half of cooked bacon to pot and stir. Click lid closed. Press the Manual button and adjust time for 4 minutes.

4. When timer beeps, quick-release the pressure. When pressure valve drops, remove lid and stir. Add in remaining bacon, cheddar, and top with chives. Serve warm.

Nutrition: Calories: 213 Protein: 9g Fiber: 6 g Fat: 30 g Sodium: 333 mg Carbohydrates: 3.3 g Sugar: 6.7 g

29. Broccoli Cheddar Dip

Preparation Time: 5 minutes

Cooking Time: 10 minutes

Servings: 6

Ingredients:

- 4 tablespoons butter
- 1/2 medium onion, diced
- 11/2 cups chopped broccoli
- 8 ounces' cream cheese
- 1/2 cup mayo
- 1/2 cup Chicken Broth (see recipe in Chapter 3)
- 1 cup shredded cheddar cheese

Directions:

1. Press the Sauté button and then press the Adjust button to set heat to Less. Add butter to Instant Pot. Add onion and sauté until softened, about 5 minutes. Press the Cancel button.

2. Add broccoli, cream cheese, mayo, and broth to pot. Press the Manual button and adjust time for 4 minutes.

3. When timer beeps, quick-release the pressure and stir in cheddar. Serve warm.

Nutrition: Calories: 321 Protein: 9 g Fiber: 1 g Fat: 29.9 g Sodium: 413 mg Carbohydrates: 4 g Sugar: 5 g

30. Hot Crab Dip

Preparation Time: 5 minutes

Cooking Time: 5 minutes

Servings: 4

Ingredients:

- 8 ounces' cream cheese
- 1 pound cooked lump crab meat
- 1/4 cup mayo
- 1/4 cup sour cream
- 1/4 teaspoon pepper
- 1/4 teaspoon salt
- 1/2 tablespoon lemon juice
- 1/2 teaspoon hot sauce
- 1/4 cup chopped pickled jalapeños
- 1/2 cup shredded cheddar
- 1/4 cup chopped green onions
- 1 cup water

Directions:

1. Place all ingredients in 7-cup glass bowl and mix. Cover with aluminum foil.

2. Pour water into Instant Pot and place steam rack in bottom. Place bowl on steam rack and click lid closed. Press the Manual button and adjust time for 5 minutes. When timer beeps, quick-release the pressure. Stir.

Nutrition: Calories: 123 Protein: 3 g Fiber: 5 g Fat: 11 g Sodium: 123 mg Carbohydrates: 5 g Sugar: 7 g

31. Creamy Chorizo Dip

Preparation Time: 5 minutes

Cooking Time: 15 minutes

Servings: 4

Ingredients:

- 1-pound ground chorizo
- 1 cup Chicken Broth
- 1/2 cup salsa
- 8 ounces' cream cheese
- 1/2 cup shredded white American cheese

Directions:

1. Press the Sauté button and add chorizo to Instant Pot. Cook thoroughly and drain or pat with paper towel to absorb grease.

2. Add broth and salsa. Place cream cheese on top of meat. Click lid closed. Press the Manual button to adjust time for 5 minutes.

3. When timer beeps, quick-release the pressure and stir in white American cheese. Serve warm.

Nutrition: Calories: 688 Protein: 28.4 g Fiber: 0.4 g Fat: 53.1 g Sodium: 1,828 mg Carbohydrates: 3 g Sugar: 2.7 g

32. Buffalo Chicken Meatballs

Preparation Time: 5 minutes

Cooking Time: 10 minutes

Servings: 4

Ingredients:

- 1-pound ground chicken
- 1/2 cup almond flour
- 2 tablespoons cream cheese
- 1 packet dry ranch dressing mix
- 1/2 teaspoon salt
- 1/4 teaspoon pepper
- 1/4 teaspoon garlic powder
- 1 cup water
- 2 tablespoons butter, melted
- 1/3 cup hot sauce
- 1/4 cup crumbled feta cheese
- 1/4 cup sliced green onion

Directions:

1. In large bowl, mix ground chicken, almond flour, cream cheese, ranch, salt, pepper, and garlic powder. Roll mixture into 16 balls.

2. Place meatballs on steam rack and add 1 cup water to Instant Pot. Click lid closed. Press the Meat button and set time for 10 minutes.

3. Combine butter and hot sauce. When timer beeps, remove meatballs and place in clean large bowl. Toss in hot sauce mixture. Top with sprinkled feta and green onions to serve.

Directions: Calories: 367 Protein: 25.0 g Fiber: 1.8 g Fat: 24.9 g Sodium: 1,131 mg Carbohydrates: 4.2 g Sugar: 1.3 g

33. Buffalo Chicken Dip

Preparation Time: 5 minutes

Cooking Time: 20 minutes

Servings: 6

Ingredients:

- 3 boneless, skinless chicken breasts
- 1 teaspoon salt
- 1/2 teaspoon garlic powder
- 1/4 teaspoon pepper
- 3/4 cup Chicken Broth (see recipe in Chapter 3)
- 1/2 cup buffalo sauce
- 4 ounces' cream cheese, softened
- 3 tablespoons butter
- 1 cup shredded cheddar cheese

Directions:

1. Place chicken breasts in Instant Pot® and sprinkle both sides with salt, garlic powder, and pepper. Add broth and buffalo sauce to pot. Click lid closed and press the Manual button to adjust time for 20 minutes.

2. When timer beeps, allow a 5-minute natural release and then quick-release the remaining pressure. Shred chicken with two forks and mix in cream cheese, butter, and cheddar.

Nutrition: Calories: 297 Protein: 25.1 g Fiber: 0.1 g Net Carbohydrates: 1.2 g Fat: 20.4 g Sodium: 1,230 mg Carbohydrates: 1.3 g Sugar: 0.7 g

34. Simple Meatballs

Preparation Time: 5 minutes

Cooking Time: 9 minutes

Servings: 4

Ingredients:

- 1-pound lean ground beef
- 1/4 cup almond flour
- 1/4 cup grated Parmesan
- 1 egg
- 2 teaspoons dried parsley
- 1 teaspoon salt
- 1/2 teaspoon dried oregano
- 1/4 teaspoon pepper
- 1 cup Easy Tomato Sauce (see recipe in this chapter)
- 1/2 cup Beef Broth (see recipe in Chapter 3)

Directions:

1. In large bowl, mix ground beef, almond flour, Parmesan, egg, parsley, salt, oregano, and pepper. Fully combine and roll into 12 balls.

2. Place tomato sauce and broth in bottom of Instant Pot®. Add meatballs, turning each one to coat in sauce. Click lid closed. Press the Manual button and adjust time for 9 minutes.

3. When timer beeps, allow a 5-minute natural release and quick-release the remaining pressure. Spoon sauce over meatballs. Serve warm.

Nutrition: Calories: 326 g Protein: 26.6 g Fiber: 2.4 g Fat: 23.4 g Sodium: 1,058 mg Carbohydrates: 3.2 grams Sugar: 4.5 g

35. **Tuna Deviled Eggs**

Preparation Time: 10 minutes

Cooking Time: 8 minutes

Servings: 3

Ingredients:

- 1 cup water
- 6 eggs
- 1 can tuna, drained
- 4 tablespoons mayo
- 1 teaspoon lemon juice
- 1 celery stalk, diced finely
- 1/4 teaspoon Dijon mustard
- 1/4 teaspoon chopped fresh dill
- 1/4 teaspoon salt
- 1/8 teaspoon garlic powder

Directions:

1. Add water to Instant Pot. Place steam rack or steamer basket inside pot. Carefully put eggs into steamer basket. Click lid closed. Press the Egg button and adjust time for 8 minutes.

2. Add remaining ingredients to medium bowl and mix.

3. When timer beeps, quick-release the steam and remove eggs. Place in bowl of cool water for 10 minutes, then remove shells.

4. Cut eggs in half and remove hard-boiled yolks, setting whites aside. Place yolks in food processor and pulse until smooth, or mash with fork. Add yolks to bowl with tuna and mayo, mixing until smooth.

5. Spoon mixture into egg-white halves. Serve chilled.

Nutrition: Calories: 303 Protein: 20.2 g Fiber: 0.2 g Fat: 22.4 g Sodium: 558 mg Carbohydrates: 1.5 g Sugar: 0.7 g

36. Avocado Egg Salad

Preparation Time: 10 minutes

Cooking Time: 8 minutes

Servings: 2

Ingredients:

- 1 cup water
- 6 eggs
- 1 avocado
- 2 tablespoons lime juice
- 1/2 teaspoon chili powder
- 1/4 teaspoon salt
- 2 tablespoons mayo
- 2 tablespoons chopped cilantro

Directions:

1. Pour water into Instant Pot. Place eggs on steam rack or in steamer basket inside pot.

2. Click lid closed. Press the Egg button and adjust time for 8 minutes. While egg is cooking, cut avocado in half and scoop out flesh. Place in food processor and blend until smooth.

3. Transfer avocado to medium bowl and add lime juice, chili powder, salt, mayo, and cilantro.

4. When timer beeps, carefully remove eggs and place in bowl of cold water for 5 minutes. Peel eggs and chop into bite-sized pieces. Fold chopped eggs into avocado mixture. Serve chilled.

Nutrition: Calories: 426 Protein: 20.5 g Fiber: 5.0 g Fat: 32.6 g Sodium: 615 mg Carbohydrates: 1.5 g Sugar: 1.2 g

VEGETABLES RECIPES

37. Keto Red Curry

Preparation Time: 20 minutes

Cooking Time: 15-20 minutes

Servings: 6

Ingredients:

- 1cup broccoli florets
- 1large handful of fresh spinach
- 4 Tbsp. coconut oil
- 1/4 medium onion
- 1 tsp. garlic, minced
- 1 tsp. fresh ginger, peeled and minced
- 2tsp. soy sauce
- 1 Tbsp. red curry paste
- 1/2 cup coconut cream

Directions:

1. Add half the coconut oil to a saucepan and heat over medium-high heat.
2. When the oil is hot, put in the onion to the pan and sauté for 3-4 minutes, until it is semi-translucent.
3. Sauté garlic, stirring, just until fragrant, about 30 seconds.
4. Lower the heat to medium-low and add broccoli florets. Sauté, stirring, for about 1-2 minutes.

5. Now, add the red curry paste. Sauté until the paste is fragrant, then mix everything.

6. Add the spinach on top of the vegetable mixture. When the spinach begins to wilt, add the coconut cream and stir.

7. Add the rest of the coconut oil, the soy sauce, and the minced ginger. Bring to a simmer for 5-10 minutes.

8. Serve hot.

Nutrition: Calories: 265 Fat: 7.1g Fiber: 6.9g Carbohydrates: 2.1 g Protein: 4.4g

38. Sweet-And-Sour Tempeh

Preparation Time: 10 minutes

Cooking Time: 25 minutes

Servings: 4

Ingredients:

- Tempeh
- 1package of tempeh
- 3/4 cup of vegetable broth
- 2tablespoons of soy sauce
- 2tablespoons olive oil
- Sauce
- 1can of pineapple juice
- 2tablespoons of brown sugar
- 1/4 cup of white vinegar
- 1 tablespoon of cornstarch
- 1 red bell pepper
- 1 chopped white onion

Directions:

1. Place a skillet on high heat. Pour in the vegetable broth and tempeh in it.

2. Add the soy sauce to the tempeh. Let it cook until it softens. This usually takes 10 minutes.

3. When it is well cooked, remove the tempeh and keep the liquid. We are going to use it for the sauce.

4. Put the tempeh in another skillet placed on medium heat.

5. Sauté it with olive oil and cook until the tempeh is browned. This should take 3 minutes.

6. Place a pot of the reserved liquid from the cooked tempeh on medium heat.

7. Add the pineapple juice, vinegar, brown sugar, and cornstarch. Stir everything together until it's well combined.

8. Let it simmer for 5 minutes.

9. Add the onion and pepper to the sauce.

10. Stir in until the sauce is thick.

11. Reduce the heat, add the cooked tempeh and pineapple chunks to the sauce. Leave it to simmer together.

12. Remove from heat and serve with any grain food of your choice.

Nutrition: Calories: 312 Fat: 10g Fiber: 4.1g Carbohydrates: 2.1 g Protein: 5.2g

39. Sherry Chicken with Mashed Potatoes

Preparation Time: 5 minutes

Cooking time: 4 hrs.

Servings: 4

Ingredients

- For the Sherry Chicken:
- 1/4 cup dry sherry
- 1cup raisins
- 4 medium-sized chicken breasts
- 1 tart cooking apple, peeled and chopped
- 1 sweet onion, sliced
- 1 cup chicken broth
- Salt and pepper, to taste
- 2pounds Idaho potatoes, peeled and cooked
- 1/4 sour cream
- 1/3 cup whole milk
- 1/2tablespoons butter
- 1 teaspoon sea salt
- 1/4 teaspoon black pepper
- 1/4 teaspoon cayenne pepper

Directions

1. In a crock pot, place all of the ingredients for the sherry chicken; cover and cook on high until chicken breasts are tender or 3 to 4 hours.

2. Meanwhile, beat potatoes, adding sour cream, milk, and butter; beat until smooth and uniform.

3. Season with spices and serve on the side with sherry chicken.

Nutrition: Calories: 154 Fat: 12 g Carbs: 3 g Protein: 15 g

40. Chicken with Zucchini

Preparation Time: 5 minutes

Cooking time: 8 hours.

Servings: 4

Ingredients

- 4 medium-sized chicken breasts, skinless
- 2 cups petite-diced tomatoes
- 1stock cube
- 1/2 cup dry white wine
- 1/2 cup water
- 1 medium zucchini, sliced
- 1 large-sized onion, chopped
- 1/3 cup fennel bulb., chopped
- 1 teaspoon ground cumin
- 1 teaspoon dried basil leaves
- 1 bay leaf
- A pinch of black pepper
- 1/4 cup olives, pitted and sliced
- 1 teaspoon lemon juice
- 2cups cooked rice

Directions

1. Place all ingredients, except olives, lemon juice and cooked rice, in a crock pot; cover and cook on low about 8 hours, adding pitted olives during last 30 minutes of cooking time.

2. Add lemon juice; discard bay leaf. Serve over cooked rice and enjoy.

Nutrition: Calories: 120 Fat: 10 g Carbs: 4 g Protein: 11 g

41. Chicken and Bell Pepper Kabobs

Preparation time: 10 minutes

Cooking time: 10 minutes

Servings: 6

Ingredients:

- 2tablespoons olive oil
- 4 tablespoons dry sherry
- 1tablespoon stone-ground mustard
- 1½ pounds (680 g) chicken, skinless, boneless and cubed
- 2red onions, cut into wedges
- 1green bell pepper, cut into 1-inch pieces
- 1red bell pepper, cut into 1-inch pieces
- 1yellow bell pepper, cut into 1-inch pieces
- ½ teaspoon sea salt
- ¼ teaspoon ground black pepper, or more to taste

Directions:

1. In a mixing bowl, combine the olive oil, dry sherry, mustard and chicken until well coated.
2. Alternate skewering the chicken and vegetables until you run out of ingredients. Season with salt and black pepper.
3. Preheat your grill to medium-high heat.
4. Place the kabobs on the grill, flipping every 2minutes and cook to desired doneness. Serve warm.

Nutrition: calories: 201 fats: 8.2g protein: 24.3g carbs:7.0 g net carbs: 5.7g fiber: 1.3g

42. Turkish Chicken Thigh Kebabs

Preparation time: 15 minutes

Cooking time: 9 to 12minutes

Servings: 2

Ingredients:

- 1pound (454 g) chicken thighs, boneless, skinless and halved
- ½ cup Greek yogurt
- Sea salt, to taste
- 1tablespoon Aleppo red pepper flakes
- ½ teaspoon ground black pepper
- ¼ teaspoon dried oregano
- ½ teaspoon mustard seeds
- 1/8 teaspoon ground cinnamon
- ½ teaspoon sumac
- 2Roma tomatoes, chopped
- 2tablespoons olive oil
- 1½ ounces (43 g) Swiss cheese, sliced

Directions:

1. Place the chicken thighs, yogurt, salt, red pepper flakes, black pepper, oregano, mustard seeds, cinnamon, sumac, tomatoes, and olive oil in a ceramic dish. Cover and let it marinate in your refrigerator for 4 hours.

2. Preheat your grill for medium-high heat and lightly oil the grate. Thread the chicken thighs onto skewers, making a thick log shape.

3. Cook your kebabs for 3 or 4 minutes; turn over and continue cooking for 3 to 4 minutes more. An instant-read thermometer should read about 165°F (74°C).

4. Add the cheese and let it cook for a further 3 to 4 minutes or until completely melted. Bon appétit!

Nutrition: calories: 500 fats: 23.3g protein: 61.0g carbs: 6.2g net carbs: 4.5g fiber: 1.7g

43. Chicken Thigh and Kale Stew

Preparation time: 20 minutes

Cooking time: 6 hours

Servings: 6

Ingredients:

- 3 tablespoons extra-virgin olive oil, divided
- 1pound (454 g) boneless chicken thighs, diced into 1½-inch pieces
- ½ sweet onion, chopped
- 2teaspoons minced garlic
- 2cups chicken broth
- 2celery stalks, diced
- 1carrot, diced
- 1teaspoon dried thyme
- 1cup shredded kale
- 1cup coconut cream
- Salt, for seasoning
- Freshly ground black pepper, for seasoning

Directions:

1. Lightly grease the insert of the slow cooker with 1tablespoon of the olive oil.

2. In a large skillet over medium-high heat, heat the remaining 2tablespoons of the olive oil. Add the chicken and sauté until it is just cooked through, about 7 minutes.

3. Add the onion and garlic and sauté for an additional 3 minutes.

4. Transfer the chicken mixture to the insert, and stir in the broth, celery, carrot, and thyme.

5. Cover and cook on low for 6 hours.

6. Stir in the kale and coconut cream.

7. Season with salt and pepper, and serve warm.

Nutrition: calories: 277 fats: 22.0g protein: 17.0g carbs: 6.0g net carbs: 4.0g fiber: 2.0g

FISH AND SEAFOOD RECIPES

44. Halibut Tacos with Cabbage Slaw

Preparation time:15 minutes

Cooking time: 6 minutes

Servings: 4

Ingredients:

- 1tablespoon olive oil
- 1teaspoon chili powder
- 4 halibut fillets, skinless, sliced
- 2low carb tortillas
- Slaw:
- 2tablespoons red cabbage, shredded
- 1tablespoon lemon juice
- Salt to taste
- ½ tablespoon extra-virgin olive oil
- ½ carrot, shredded
- 1tablespoon cilantro, chopped

Directions:

1. Combine red cabbage with salt in a bowl; massage cabbage to tenderize. Add in the remaining slaw ingredient, toss to coat and set aside.

2. Rub the halibut with olive oil, chili powder and paprika. Heat a grill pan over medium heat.

3. Add halibut and cook until lightly charred and cooked through, about 3 minutes per side.

4. Divide between the tortillas. Combine all slaw ingredients in a bowl. Split the slaw among the tortillas.

Nutrition: calories: 386 fats: 25.9g protein: 23.7g carbs: 12.6g net carbs: 6.4g fiber: 6.2g

45. Coconut Shrimp Stew

Preparation time:15 minutes

Cooking time: 15 minutes

Servings: 6

Ingredients:

- 1cup coconut milk
- 2tablespoons lime juice
- ¼ cup diced roasted peppers
- 1½ pounds (680 g) shrimp, peeled and deveined
- ¼ cup olive oil
- 1garlic clove, minced
- 14 ounces (397 g) diced tomatoes
- 2tablespoons sriracha sauce
- ¼ cup onions, chopped
- ¼ cup cilantro, chopped
- Fresh dill, chopped to garnish
- Salt and black pepper to taste

Directions:

1. Heat the olive oil in a pot over medium heat. Add onions and, cook for 3 minutes, or until translucent.

2. Add the garlic and cook, for another minute, until soft. Add tomatoes, shrimp, and cilantro. Cook until the shrimp becomes opaque, about 3-4 minutes. Stir in sriracha and coconut milk, and cook, for 2more minutes. Do NOT bring to a boil. Stir in the lime juice, and season with salt and pepper to taste. Spoon the stew in bowls, garnish with fresh dill, and serve warm.

Nutrition: calories: 325 fats: 20.9g protein: 22.8g carbs: 6.2g net carbs: 5.1g fiber: 1.1g

46. Asparagus and Trout Foil Packets

Preparation time: 15 minutes

Cooking time: 15 minutes

Servings: 4

Ingredients:

- 1pound (454 g) asparagus spears
- 1tablespoon garlic purée
- 1pound (454 g) deboned trout, butterflied
- Salt and black pepper to taste
- 3 tablespoons olive oil
- 2sprigs rosemary
- 2sprigs thyme
- 2tablespoons butter
- ½ medium red onion, sliced
- 2lemon slices

Directions:

1. Preheat the oven to 400°F (205°C). Rub the trout with garlic purée, salt and black pepper.

2. Prepare two aluminum foil squares. Place the fish on each square. Divide the asparagus and onion between the squares, top with a pinch of salt and pepper, a sprig of rosemary and thyme, and 1tablespoon of butter. Also, lay the lemon slices on the fish. Wrap and close the fish packets securely, and place them on a baking sheet. Bake in the oven for 15 minutes, and remove once ready.

Nutrition: calories: 495 fats: 39.2g protein: 26.9g carbs: 7.5g net carbs: 4.9g fiber: 2.6g

SALADS RECIPES

47. Zucchini and Bell Pepper Slaw

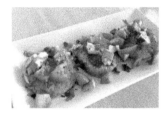

Preparation time: 15 minutes

Cooking time: 0 minutes

Servings: 3

Ingredients:

- 1zucchini, shredded
- 1yellow bell pepper, sliced
- 1red onion, thinly sliced
- 2tablespoons extra-virgin olive oil
- 1tablespoon balsamic vinegar
- 1teaspoon Dijon mustard
- ¼ teaspoon cumin seeds
- ¼ teaspoon ground black pepper
- Sea salt, to taste

Directions:

1. Thoroughly combine all ingredients in a salad bowl.
2. Refrigerate for 1hour before serving or serve right away. Enjoy!

Nutrition: calories: 97 fat: 9.5g protein: 0.8g carbs: 2.7g net carbs: 2.4g fiber: 0.3g

48. Bell Pepper, Cabbage, and Arugula Coleslaw

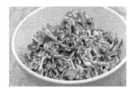

Preparation time: 15 minutes

Cooking time: 0 minutes

Servings: 4

Ingredients:

- 2teaspoons balsamic vinegar
- 1teaspoon fresh garlic, minced
- 2tablespoons tahini (sesame paste)
- 1tablespoon yellow mustard
- Sea salt and ground black pepper, to taste
- ¼ teaspoon paprika
- 1red bell pepper, deveined and sliced
- 1green bell pepper, deveined and sliced
- ½ pound (227 g) Napa cabbage, shredded
- 2cups arugula, torn into pieces
- 1Spanish onion, thinly sliced into rings
- 4 tablespoons sesame seeds, lightly toasted

Directions:

1. Make a dressing by whisking the balsamic vinegar, garlic, tahini, mustard, salt, black pepper, and paprika.

2. In a salad bowl, combine the bell peppers, cabbage, arugula, and Spanish onion. Dress the salad and toss until everything is well incorporated.

3. Garnish with sesame seeds just before serving. Serve well chilled and enjoy!

Nutrition: calories: 123 fat: 9.2g protein: 4.6g carbs: 5.8g net carbs: 2.8g fiber: 3.0g

DESSERT

49. No Bake Low Carb Lemon Strawberry Cheesecake

Preparation Time: 15 Minutes

Cooking Time: 45 minutes

Servings: 2

Ingredients:

- 1/2cup cream cheese
- 2teaspoons of lemon extract
- 3/4 cup heavy whipped cream
- Zest of 1lemon
- 1/3 cup sweetener
- 2big strawberries

Directions:

1. Add cream cheese, sweetener, and whipped cream in a bowl. Beat it at high speed until smooth and creamy. Add lemon extract and mix. Take 1strawberry and chop it into small pieces. Cut the other strawberry in the shape of a heart.

2. Fill half of each jar with half of the cream cheese mixture. Add the chopped strawberry to the jars to get a nice layer. Cover the strawberries with the rest of the cream cheese mixture.

3. Use the strawberry slices to create a flow pattern on top. Sprinkle with lemon zest in the center of each flower. Cool in refrigerator. Your dessert is ready

Nutrition: Calories 365 Fat 12 Fiber 1.9 Carbs 3.8 Protein 7

50. Pecan Cheesecake

Preparation Time: 15 Minutes

Cooking Time: 40 minutes

Servings: 12

Ingredients:

- 2cups of almond flour
- 2eggs
- 3 tablespoons of butter
- 8 oz. / 1cup cream cheese
- 1/2teaspoon vanilla
- 1/2- 1teaspoon maple extract
- 1cup sugar Swerve
- 1cup pecans and 2tablespoons for garnishing

Directions:

1. Melt butter and mix with flour, vanilla, and swerve. Stir in the egg yolk (1egg). Insert in a tart pan by pressing with your fingers. Bake for 10 minutes at 180 degrees C. Mix Cream cheese with vanilla, maple extract, and eggs.

2. Chop pecans. Mix with a little sea salt. Put the pecans first. Pour cheesecake mixture. Garnish with two tablespoons of pecans.

3. Bake for 20 minutes at 170 degrees C or until the cream cheese mixture is set. Cool completely.

4. Cool for at least six hours, preferably overnight. Cut into 16 squares.

Nutrition: Calories 123 Fat 11 Fiber 4 Carbs 4 Protein 17

CONCLUSION

The keto diet is a special type of diet that drastically lowers your carbohydrate intake and replaces it with fats. When you're in ketosis, your body enters into a metabolic state where most of the energy comes from ketones, which are produced by the liver as well as being broken down in fat cells. Ketosis has some pretty great benefits: it can help you lose weight without feeling ravenous all the time, it can help you clear up acne and other skin problems, and more! The catch? You have to be willing to cut out or eliminate many types of food from your diet.

What Can You Eat?

Most of the foods you eat on a keto diet are high in fat. Most types of meats are off-limits, except for fatty cuts like beef chuck steak, ground pork belly, bacon and fatback. Dairy is also out, with the exception of heavy cream and cheese made from full-fat milk. Eggs are fine to consume – it's when you start adding other animal products that things can get dicey.

The main types of food you'll eat on a ketogenic diet are dairy foods, fish, meat and eggs. Some people also like to consume vegetables that are relatively low in carbs, like leafy greens or cruciferous vegetables.

Sugars: Your New Enemy… Or Not?

Maybe you've heard that sugar is bad for your health and people have been warning you about it for years. Well… It's true! When you eat a lot of sugar, sugar molecules can attach themselves to proteins in your body and become glycated. Glycated proteins can go on to do some serious damage to your arteries as well as causing inflammation. They can also lead to the onset of many types of diseases, and that's why it's important to avoid them – but is this really possible on a keto diet?

Some people say that all sugars must be eliminated from a keto diet because they will immediately be transformed into glycated proteins.

However, this isn't entirely accurate. While it's true that there are many processes in the body that can turn sugars into toxic glycated proteins, this doesn't happen when you eat natural sugar from fruits, starchy foods or even your favorite fruit salad. The main problem is that refined sugars and their byproducts are not part of the keto diet plan.

Furthermore, since a significant amount of carbohydrates on a ketogenic diet come from sugar alcohols (think mannitol and lactitol), many people prefer to limit or eliminate those in their diets as well. The final caveat is that if you're looking to lose fat fast, avoid any form of sugar at all costs – including natural ones! Choose natural sweeteners like Stevia instead.

What About Sugar Alcohols?

In addition to being high in calories, sugars from sugar alcohols are also difficult for the body to process. This is one of the main reasons why they've become so popular as diet foods. Though they have fewer calories than regular sugar and carbohydrates, these types of sugar still cause an overload of glucose in your body – which can lead to insulin resistance and weight gain.

While some types of sugar alcohols don't have as many calories per gram as others, they still pack a lot of calories into just a few teaspoons. For instance, one teaspoon of Mannitol has 24 calories. Xylitol only has about 13 calories per teaspoon, but that still adds up.

Because ketogenic diets remove most carbohydrates and sugars from the diet and limit fats to under 70% of total caloric intake, eating too much sugar alcohol can prevent you from reaching ketosis.

Lightning Source UK Ltd.
Milton Keynes UK
UKHW021832200421
382338UK00003B/300